Diy Red Light Therapy

A Natural Approach to Health and Healing

Fredric Clark

Red Light Therapy
Definition Red light therapy

Red light therapy (RLT) is a type of medicine that penetrates the skin to provide a number of health benefits by using particular red and near-infrared light wavelengths. This therapy uses low-level lasers or light-emitting diodes (LEDs) to give light energy to the body's tissues, which can promote healing processes, lower inflammation, and improve cellular function. RLT is a non-invasive, painless, and all-natural method of enhancing general health and wellbeing. Its uses

range from pain treatment and
skin renewal to wound healing
and mental health enhancement.

Chapter One

Natural methods are important for health

The holistic and frequently non-invasive nature of natural approaches to health makes them valuable alternatives that can either supplement or completely replace traditional medical therapies. The following are some salient points emphasizing their importance:

1. Reduced Adverse Reactions:

• In general, side effects from natural therapies are lower than those from pharmaceuticals and invasive medical procedures.

Patients may have a higher quality of life as a result of fewer negative effects.

2. Enhances General Well-Being:

• Treating the full person rather than simply the disease's symptoms is a common goal of natural therapies. Enhancements in one's physical, mental, and emotional well-being can result from adopting this holistic viewpoint.

3. Encourages Preventive Healthcare:

• A lot of natural remedies, like healthy eating, consistent

exercise, and stress reduction
methods, are preventive in
nature. They can aid in
preserving health and delaying
the emergence of long-term
illnesses.

4. Encourages Patients:

• Patients are frequently
encouraged to actively participate
in their own health and well-being
by natural health approaches.
Increased adherence to good
lifestyle choices and a stronger
sense of control over one's health
might result from this
empowerment.

5. Economical:

• Compared to traditional medical treatments, many natural health activities, such as exercise, mindfulness, and dietary adjustments, can be more affordable. In particular, this can help with long-term health condition management.

6. Both accessible and sustainable:

Why A greater populace can access natural ways because they frequently make use of sustainable and easily accessible resources. In places where access to cutting-edge medical care is scarce, this accessibility may be vital.

7. Supplemental to Traditional Medical Care:

• To increase the efficacy of conventional treatments and lessen reliance on prescription drugs, natural therapies can be used in conjunction with them. Integrative medicine is becoming more and more well-known for its all-encompassing care, as it integrates both methods.

8. Pay Attention to the Causes:

• Rather than just treating symptoms, natural health

methods seek to address the underlying causes of health problems. This may result in longer-lasting and more potent treatments for persistent illnesses.

9. Boosts the Processes of Natural Healing:

• A lot of natural treatments strengthen and assist the body's natural healing processes. The body's natural healing and regeneration processes, for instance, can be stimulated by treatments like herbal medicine, acupuncture, and red light therapy.

10. Lessens Stress and Promotes Mental Wellness:

• Natural strategies like yoga, meditation, and mindfulness can lower stress and enhance mental health, promoting general wellbeing and resiliency to disease.

Chapter Three

Explanation of Wavelengths in Red Light Therapy

Using particular light wavelengths, particularly in the red and near-infrared (NIR) spectrum, is known as red light treatment (RLT). These wavelengths, which are expressed in nanometers (nm), normally fall between 600 and 1000 nm. Below is an explanation of certain wavelengths' functions and advantages:

Dark Red (600–700 nm)

• **Penetration Depth:** Around 8 to 10 millimeters are how deep red light in this range may penetrate skin.

- **Cellular Benefits:** This wavelength stimulates cellular activity, increases the generation of ATP (adenosine triphosphate), and promotes the synthesis of collagen by being absorbed by the skin and surface tissues.

- **Advantages:**

- **Skin Health:** Enhances the texture and tone of the skin, minimizes fine lines and wrinkles, and speeds up the healing of wounds.

- **Inflammation Reduction:**
Aids in the healing of minor
injuries by reducing inflammation.

Light in the near-infrared (700–
1000 nm)

- **Penetration Depth:** NIR light
may reach muscles, joints, and
even bones by penetrating tissues
at a deeper depth.

- **Cellular Benefits:** Because
NIR wavelengths can reach
deeper tissues, they can improve
cellular regeneration and repair
as well as blood circulation and
inflammation reduction.

- **Advantages:**

- **Pain Relief**: Helps with ailments including arthritis and muscle injuries by reducing pain and inflammation in deeper tissues.

- **Enhanced Recovery:** Promotes muscular recuperation and shortens the healing period following physical strain or injury.

- **General Health:** Enhances immune system support, encourages tissue healing, and enhances general cell function.

Chapter Four

How Red light Therapy works

Red light treatment (RLT) stimulates cellular activity and offers a range of therapeutic advantages by penetrating the skin and tissues with particular light wavelengths. Here's a thorough examination of the RLT's workings:

1. Light Penetration

• Red light (600–700 nm): Affects the dermis and epidermis after penetrating the skin to a depth of 8–10 millimeters.

• Near-infrared light (700–1000 nm): This type of light can

penetrate up to several centimeters into tissues, including muscles, joints, and bones.

2. Intake by Cellular Component

• **Chromophores:** Red and near-infrared light are absorbed by certain chemicals found in cells called chromophores. The mitochondrial enzyme cytochrome c oxidase is one of the main chromophores.

3. Stimulation of Mitochondria

• **Greater Production of ATP:** Chromophore absorption causes the mitochondria, the cell's energy factory, to make more

ATP (adenosine triphosphate), the unit of account for energy in the cell. Increased ATP synthesis increases metabolism and cellular energy.

• Improved Cellular perform: When there is more ATP available, cells are able to repair damage, regenerate, and perform more effectively.

4. Diminution of Oxidative Damage

• Reactive Oxygen Species (ROS): RLT balances the generation of ROS and strengthens antioxidant defenses, which helps to reduce oxidative stress. This decrease in oxidative stress promotes general cellular health and shields cells from harm.

5. Adjustment of Inflammation

• Anti-Inflammatory Effects: RLT decreases pro-inflammatory cytokine levels and increases anti-inflammatory cytokine synthesis in order to control the inflammatory response. This aids in reducing swelling and encouraging recovery.

6. Enhanced Blood Circulation

• Vasodilation: RLT stimulates blood vessel enlargement, or vasodilation, which enhances blood flow. Improved oxygen and nutrition supply to tissues through increased blood flow promotes healing and recovery.

7. Production of Collagen

• Fibroblast Stimulation: RLT activates fibroblasts, which are the cells that make collagen. More collagen is produced, which increases wound healing, minimizes wrinkles, and enhances skin flexibility.

Important Mechanisms in Action

1. Enhanced Production of ATP:

• The absorption of light energy by mitochondria increases the creation of ATP, giving cells greater energy to carry out their tasks efficiently.

2. Improved Cellular Regeneration and Repair:

• Faster cell and tissue regeneration and repair is made possible by higher ATP levels, which aid in healing and recuperation.

3. Reducing Inflammation:

• RLT helps to ease pain and promote healing by reducing inflammation through modifying cytokine levels.

4. Enhanced Circulation and Blood Flow:

• Improved circulation guarantees that tissues receive oxygen and nutrients more effectively, supporting tissue growth and repair.

5. Synthesis of Collagen:

• Increasing the production of collagen strengthens the skin, minimizes aging symptoms, and hastens the healing of cuts and scars.

Practical Applications

• **Skin rejuvenation** improves the texture and tone of the skin, minimizes wrinkles, and speeds up the healing of scars and acne.

• **Discomfort relief:** lessens inflammation, eases discomfort in the joints and muscles, and aids in the healing process following injuries.

• **Mental Health:** Enhances energy and mood, which may help people who suffer from seasonal affective disorder (SAD), anxiety, or sadness.

• **Wound Healing:** Reduces the production of scars and speeds up the healing of burns, cuts, and wounds.

Chapter Five

Types of device used in Red Light Therapy

Red light treatment (RLT) equipment is available in a variety of shapes and sizes, each intended to meet specific requirements. Light-emitting diodes (LEDs) or low-level lasers are the main sources of light used by these gadgets to provide red and near-infrared light to the body. The primary kinds of RLT devices are as follows:

1. LED Displays

• Description: Red and near-infrared light is emitted by large panels fitted with numerous LEDs.

• Usage: Frequently used for treatments involving the entire body or for larger areas like the legs or back.

• Benefits: They are effective for whole-body therapy since they can treat large areas in a single session.

2. Portable Electronics

• Description: Handheld, tiny, LED-equipped gadgets that are portable and can be moved throughout the body.

• Usage: Perfect for focusing on particular regions, such the joints, face, or specific pain locations.

• Advantages: Exceptionally practical and user-friendly, ideal for both home and travel use.

3. Masks for Light Therapy

• Description: LED-embedded face masks made especially for facial care procedures.

• Usage: Mainly used for skin health, such as skin regeneration, acne treatment, and anti-aging.

• Benefits: Offers uniform coverage for the skin on the face, improving treatment efficacy.

4. Beds for Light Therapy

• Description: Full-body beds that resemble tanning beds but don't emit UV light due to their abundance of LEDs.

• Usage: Applied to complete full-body therapy in clinical or spa settings.

• Advantages: Provides consistent exposure to red light throughout the body, enhancing general health and wellbeing.

5. Laser Equipment

• Description: LEDs are replaced by focused laser beams in low-level laser therapy (LLLT) devices.

• Usage: Usually applied in medical settings for targeted therapies like pain management, wound healing, and certain therapeutic uses.

• Advantages: Provides more concentrated light radiation, which is advantageous when treating deep tissue.

6. Wearable Technology

• Description: Wearable accessories having LEDs incorporated, such as belts, pads, or wraps.

• Application: Applied to particular body regions, such as the shoulders, knees, or lower back, for targeted therapy.

• Advantages: Offers ongoing care while preserving mobility;

ideal for treating persistent pain or inflammation.

7. Combination Equipment

• Description: Red light devices that work in conjunction with other therapies, such heat therapy or blue light therapy for acne.

• Usage: Applied to diverse skin problems to improve therapeutic outcomes or as part of multimodal therapy.

• Advantages: Provides a flexible therapy method, meeting several needs with a single gadget.

Chapter Six

Important Things to Think About When Selecting a Device

1. The reason for using

• Choose whether the gadget will be used for general wellbeing, pain management, wound healing, or skin rejuvenation.

2. Treatment Area:

• Select the type and size of device according to the area that has to be treated. Think about beds or panels for larger spaces; wearable or portable electronics work best for smaller places.

3. Wavelength and Intensity:

• Verify that the device emits
light at the right wavelengths
(usually between 600 and 1000
nm) and at a strong enough
intensity to have the intended
therapeutic effect.

4. Convenience and Portability:

• While larger panels and beds
could be better suited for clinical
or professional settings, handheld
and wearable technology is more
convenient and appropriate for
usage at home.

5. Certification and Safety:

• To guarantee effectiveness and
safety, look for gadgets that are

FDA-approved or have other pertinent certifications.

6. Budget:

• Evaluate the device's price in relation to its features and advantages. While larger panels and beds can be more expensive but offer more coverage, handheld devices are typically more affordable.

Users can choose the best red light treatment equipment to suit their demands for health and wellness by being aware of the various types available and the applications for which they are best suited.

Chapter Seven

Advantages of Red Light Therapy for Health

Clinical investigations and scientific research support the many health benefits of red light therapy (RLT). a few of the main advantages:

1. Skin Wellness and Revitalization

• **Collagen Production:** RLT induces fibroblasts to produce more collagen, which enhances skin suppleness and lessens the visibility of wrinkles and fine lines.

- **Anti-Aging Effects:** Skin appears younger by improving texture and tone, minimizing pores, and reducing pigmentation.

- **Acne Treatment:** Lowers bacterial growth and irritation, aiding in the clearing of acne and averting subsequent outbreaks.

- **Scar Reduction:** Encourages quicker healing and lessens the visibility of scars, such as surgical and acne scars.

2. Reduction of Pain and Inflammation

- **Joint Pain and Arthritis:** By lowering inflammation and enhancing joint function, this treatment relieves pain and stiffness associated with diseases like rheumatoid arthritis and osteoarthritis.

● **Muscle Recovery:** By increasing blood flow and lowering inflammation, this technique improves muscle recovery and lessens discomfort following physical activity.

● **Chronic Pain Management:** By reducing inflammatory response and encouraging tissue healing, this approach helps control chronic pain problems like tendinitis and fibromyalgia.

3. Mental Well-Being and Mood Improvement

- **Seasonal Affective Disorder (SAD):** During the winter, when there is less natural sunlight, SAD symptoms are alleviated by elevating mood and vigor.

- **Anxiety and Depression:** May lessen anxiety and depression symptoms by encouraging relaxation and a sense of well-being.

4. Healing Wounds and Tissue Restoration

- **Enhanced Healing:** By encouraging cellular repair and regeneration, this treatment expedites the healing of burns, wounds, and surgical incisions.

• **Less Scarring:** Promotes the body's natural healing process and enhances collagen synthesis to reduce the creation of scars.

5. Enhanced Circulation of Blood

• **Vasodilation:** Encourages blood vessels to expand, which improves blood flow and oxygen delivery to tissues. Overall tissue health and function are supported by this improved circulation.

• **Cardiovascular Health:** By enhancing endothelial function and lowering oxidative stress, this intervention may promote cardiovascular health.

6. Reduced Inflammation Impact

- **Chronic Inflammation:** By regulating cytokine levels and boosting antioxidant defenses, this treatment reduces chronic inflammation linked to a number of illnesses, including autoimmune diseases and chronic pain syndromes.

7. Health and Hair Growth

- **Alopecia Treatment:** In cases of androgenic alopecia (male and female pattern baldness), this treatment stimulates hair follicles and encourages hair growth.

• **Hair Thickness:** By promoting the health and functionality of hair follicles, this treatment improves hair density and thickness.

8. Improved sleep quality

• Melatonin Production: Research suggests that RLT may increase melatonin production, which would improve circadian rhythm regulation and the quality of sleep.

Red light therapy is beneficial for certain conditions.

• **Eczema and psoriasis**: Encourages the healing of skin damaged by eczema and psoriasis by reducing inflammation.

• **Bursitis and tendinitis:** Promotes a quicker recovery by reducing pain and inflammation in bursae and tendons.

• **Neuropathy:** In peripheral neuropathy, which is frequently linked to chemotherapy or diabetes, it lessens pain and enhances nerve function.

• **Dental health:** expedites recovery following dental operations, lessens pain, and encourages the healing of oral tissues.

Mechanisms That Underlie the Advantages

1. Increased Cellular Energy:

• RLT promotes the synthesis of ATP in cells, giving them more energy for internal operations and improving general cell performance.

2. Decrease in Oxidative Stress

• Reactive oxygen species (ROS) generation and antioxidant

defenses are balanced by RLT, which promotes cellular health and helps shield cells from harm.

3. Improved Airflow:

• Better oxygen and nutrient delivery to tissues through increased blood flow promotes healing and lowers inflammation.

4. The anti-inflammatory reaction

• RLT promotes tissue healing by regulating the synthesis of inflammatory cytokines, which lowers inflammation.

5. Synthesis of Collagen:

• Higher collagen synthesis promotes healthy skin, lessens

scarring, and quickens the healing of wounds.

Red light therapy for acne and scar treatment

Because red light therapy (RLT) can reduce inflammation, encourage healing, and stimulate the creation of collagen, it has been shown to be beneficial in treating acne scars as well as acne. An extensive examination of how RLT can benefit several skin disorders is provided below:

Acne Treatment

1. Reducing Inflammation:

• **Inflammation Reduction:** By regulating the synthesis of inflammatory cytokines, RLT helps lessen the inflammation linked to acne. This results in decreased redness and swelling, which lessens the visibility and discomfort of existing acne.

2. Lowering of Bacteria:

• Targeting Acne-Causing Bacteria: Red light treatment can assist by lowering the total bacterial load and bolstering the immune system's response to infections, even though blue light therapy is more frequently employed to target the Propionibacterium acnes bacteria that cause acne.

3. Control of Sebum:

• Balancing Oil Production: RLT can assist in controlling the skin's sebum (oil) production, which lowers the risk of blocked pores and the development of new acne lesions.

4. Restoring Active Lesions:

• Quicker Recovery: RLT speeds up the healing of active acne lesions by encouraging cellular regeneration and repair, which lowers the chance of hyper-pigmentation and scarring.

Treatment of Scars

1. Production of Collagen:

• **Fibroblast Stimulation:** RLT encourages the skin's fibroblasts to create more collagen, which is necessary for skin restoration and the appearance of less scars. Over time, acne scars become less apparent as a result of more collagen filling them in.

2. Enhancing the Texture of Skin:

- **Smoothing Out Skin:** By lessening the roughness connected with scar tissue, regular usage of RLT helps smooth out and even out the texture of the skin.

3. Cut Down on Hyper-pigmentation

- **Evening Skin Tone:** Post-inflammatory hyper-pigmentation (PIH), which frequently coexists with acne scars, can be lessened with RLT. It aids in balancing out skin tone and lightening acne-related dark spots.

4. Reduce the Formation of Scars:

- **Prevention:** RLT lessens the chance of new scars forming by hastening the healing of active acne lesions, especially when applied early in the course of acne treatment.

Chapter Eight

Red light therapy for pain relief and inflammation reduction

The ability of red light treatment (RLT) to lessen inflammation and relieve pain is well known. People with a variety of ailments, such as chronic pain, muscle injuries, and arthritis, can benefit from this non-invasive treatment. Here's a thorough examination of how RLT reduces inflammation and eases pain:

Mechanisms of Action

1. Enhanced Energy in Cells:

• **ATP Production:** RLT increases cells' synthesis of ATP

(adenosine triphosphate), giving them more energy to carry out their daily tasks. Increased cellular energy makes it possible for injured tissues to heal and regenerate more quickly.

2. Decrease in Oxidative Stress

- **Antioxidant Effects:** RLT strengthens antioxidant defenses and assists in regulating the generation of reactive oxygen species (ROS). This decrease in oxidative stress shields cells from harm and promotes the general health of cells.

3. The anti-inflammatory reaction

• **RLT Modulates Inflammatory Cytokine Production:** It decreases pro-inflammatory cytokine levels while elevating anti-inflammatory cytokines. This aids in reducing pain and inflammation brought on by a number of ailments.

4. A better flow of blood:

• **Vasodilation:** RLT encourages blood vessel enlargement, which enhances blood flow and the supply of oxygen to tissues. Improved circulation eases pain, lowers inflammation, and aids in tissue healing.

5. Modulation of Nerve Function:

- **Pain Signal Reduction:** RLT has the ability to alter nerve function, which lessens the amount of pain signals that reach the brain and relieves chronic pain.

Red light therapy: A Useful Treatment for Pain and Inflammation

1.Duration and Frequency:

- **Treatment Sessions:**

Depending on the severity of the problem, RLT should be utilized three to five times a week for optimum outcomes. Each session should last between ten and twenty minutes.

- **Consistency:** To achieve long-term pain relief and inflammation reduction, regular and continuous use is essential.

2. Selection of Device:

• Handheld devices: These can be used to target certain pain points, like muscles or joints.

• **LED Panels:** Perfect for addressing several locations at once or bigger regions.

• **Wearable devices:** useful for chronic illnesses, they allow for mobility while providing convenient ongoing therapy.

3. Getting ready:

• **Clean Skin:** To enable the best possible light penetration, make sure the skin is clear of oils or lotions prior to treatment.

4. Following Treatment:

- **Hydration:** To promote general health and aid in the healing process, sip lots of water.
- **Pain Management:** For maximum effects, combine RLT with other pain-reduction methods including massage, stretching, or physical therapy.

Expected Result

- **Short-Term:** Better mobility and function in the treated areas, as well as an instant decrease in pain and inflammation.
- **Long-Term:** Significant reduction in the need for painkillers, significant improvement in quality of life, and less chronic pain. It can take several weeks to months of

consistent use to get noticeable
and long-lasting effects.

Chapter Nine

Red light therapy applications for arthritis and joint pain

Because red light therapy (RLT) contains anti-inflammatory and pain-relieving qualities, it has demonstrated great promise in controlling symptoms of arthritis and joint pain. RLT can be specifically used to treat arthritis and joint pain in the following ways:

Mechanisms of Action in Arthritis and Joint Pain

1.Reducing Inflammation:

• **Cytokine Modulation**: RLT decreases the synthesis of pro-inflammatory cytokines and enhances the production of anti-inflammatory cytokines, which contributes to a reduction in joint inflammation overall.

2. A better flow of blood:

• **Vasodilation:** Promotes healing and lessens stiffness by increasing blood flow to injured joints, supplying more oxygen and nutrients.

3. Reduction of Pain Signals:

• **Nerve Function Modulation:** This reduces the amount of pain signals that are sent from the joints to the brain by altering nerve activity.

4. Repairing Cartilage:

• Cellular regeneration: Promotes the development of chondrocytes, which are cells that produce cartilage, helping to preserve and repair joint cartilage.

5. Enhanced Energy in Cells:

• **ATP Production:** Increases the amount of ATP produced by cells, giving them more energy to repair themselves and less joint wear and tear.

Applications for Various Arthritis Types

1.Osteoarthritis:

• Pain Relief: By lowering inflammation and enhancing joint function, RLT relieves osteoarthritis-related pain.

• Cartilage Support: Decreases joint cartilage deterioration and encourages cartilage repair, which slows the advancement of osteoarthritis.

2. Diabetic arthritis:

• Immune modulation: lessens the autoimmune assault on joint tissues by assisting in the modulation of the immune response.

• Inflammation Reduction: This lessens swelling and pain by lowering inflammation in the synovial membrane that lines the joints.

3. Arthritis Psoriatica:

• Benefits for the Skin and Joints: Reduces inflammation and pain in the joints while also treating psoriasis-related skin lesions.

4. Gout

• Uric Acid Reduction: May assist in lowering uric acid levels in the joints, thereby reducing gout-related discomfort and inflammation.

Red light therapy: A Useful Treatment for Arthritis and Joint Pain

1.Treatment Duration and Frequency:

• **First Phase:** During the first two to three weeks, RLT can be taken daily or every other day for acute pain and inflammation.

• **Maintenance Phase:** To sustain advantages following the first phase, treatments can be cut back to two to three times per week.

2. Selection of Device:

• **Handheld devices:** Good for focusing on certain joints, like the hands, elbows, or knees.

• **LED Mats or Panels:** Ideal for treating several joints at once or bigger regions.

• **Wearable devices:** These are useful for treating afflicted joints continuously; examples include knee and elbow wraps.

3. Getting Ready and Using It:

• **Clean Skin:** Prior to receiving therapy, make sure the skin surrounding the afflicted joint is clear of any oils or lotions.

• **Direct Exposure:** For the best light penetration, place the device directly over the joint while maintaining the required distance.

4. Following Treatment:

- **Hydration:** To aid in the body's healing processes, consume lots of water.

- **Physical Activity:** To preserve joint strength and mobility, do mild exercises or stretches.

Expected Result

- **Short-Term:** Reduced swelling in the treated areas, enhanced joint mobility, and instantaneous pain and stiffness reduction.

- **Long-Term:** Decreased dependency on painkillers, enhanced joint function, and a notable reduction in chronic pain. Additionally, long-term use can enhance general joint health and decrease the advancement of arthritis.

Clinical Evidence and Case Studies

1.Osteoarthritis:

• RLT dramatically reduced pain and disability in patients with knee osteoarthritis when compared to placebo treatments, according to a study published in "Lasers in Medical Science".

2. Diabetic arthritis:

• A study that was published in "Photomedicine and Laser Surgery" showed that RLT helped rheumatoid arthritis patients with their pain and stiffness in the morning.

3. Joint Pain generally:

• A systematic review published in "Pain Research and Management" found that RLT helps with a variety of musculoskeletal diseases, including joint pain, by lowering pain and enhancing function.

Chapter Ten

Red Light Therapy for Sports Injuries and Muscle Recuperation

Athletes and fitness enthusiasts are using red light therapy (RLT) more frequently to improve muscle recovery and treat sports injuries. The therapy is a useful tool for maximizing sports performance and recovery because of its capacity to lower inflammation, relieve pain, and encourage healing. RLT can be used for sports injuries and muscle recovery in the following ways:

Mechanisms of Action for Sports Injuries and Muscle Recovery

1.Enhanced Production of Cellular Energy:

• ATP Synthesis: RLT increases muscle cells' synthesis of ATP (adenosine triphosphate), which gives cells more energy and expedites healing.

2. Diminishing Oxidative Stress:

• Antioxidant Effects: By regulating reactive oxygen species (ROS) and boosting antioxidant defenses, RLT helps lower oxidative stress. This quickens the mending process and shields muscle cells from harm.

3. Reducing Inflammation:

• Cytokine Modulation: RLT decreases muscle tissue inflammation and expedites the healing process from injuries by regulating the synthesis of pro- and anti-inflammatory cytokines.

4. Enhanced Circulation and Blood Flow:

• Vasodilation: Encourages vasodilation, which enhances blood flow to wounded tissues and muscles. Increased oxygen and nutrition delivery from improved circulation promotes healing and lessens pain in the muscles.

5. Production of Collagen:

• Tissue Repair: RLT promotes the synthesis of collagen, which is essential for the repair of muscles and connective tissue and speeds up the healing of wounds.

6. Pain Management:

• Nerve Modulation: RLT has the ability to modify nerve activity, which lessens the transmission of pain signals and relieves aches in the muscles and joints.

Uses for Recovering Muscle

1.Muscle Soreness Following Exercise:

• **Delayed Onset Muscle Soreness (DOMS):** RLT aids in lessening the intensity and length of DOMS, enabling a quicker return to exercise and enhanced function.

2. Tired Muscles:

• **Enhanced Recovery:** RLT improves overall recovery and lessens muscle fatigue by lowering inflammation and raising ATP production. This allows for more frequent training and intense sessions.

3. Strength and Muscle Growth:

• **Performance Enhancement:** By speeding up recovery and lowering the chance of overtraining injuries, regular use of RLT can promote strength and muscle growth.

Sports Injury Applications

1. Strains and Sprain:

• Accelerated Healing: By boosting cellular repair processes and lowering inflammation, RLT helps sprains and strains of the muscles heal more quickly.

2. Bursitis and tendinitis:

• Inflammation Reduction: RLT relieves pain and speeds up healing in illnesses like tendinitis and bursitis by reducing inflammation in tendons and bursae.

3. Breaks and Abrasions:

• Bone and Soft Tissue Repair: By promoting collagen synthesis and enhancing blood flow to the afflicted areas, RLT can help soft tissue injuries and fractures recover.

4. Cartilage and Ligament Injuries:

• Tissue Regeneration:
Promotes ligament and cartilage tissue regeneration, aiding in the healing of injuries including meniscus damage and ACL tears.

Use of Red Light Therapy in Practice for Sports Injuries and Muscle Recuperation

1.Treatment Duration and Frequency:

• First Phase: During the first one to two weeks, RLT can be used daily or every other day for acute injuries or post-exercise rehabilitation.

• Maintenance Phase: To sustain

the benefits of recuperation and promote continued muscular health, sessions can be cut back to once or twice a week after the initial phase.

2. Selection of Device:

• Handheld devices: Good for concentrating on injured areas or certain muscle groups.

• LED Mats or Panels: Ideal for treating numerous muscle groups or bigger areas at once.

• Wearable devices: These are useful for treating certain areas continuously, including elbow sleeves or knee wraps.

3. Getting Ready and Using It:

• Clean Skin: To allow for the best possible light penetration, make sure the skin over the injured or targeted muscle is free of oils and lotions.

• Direct Exposure: Hold the gadget directly over the impacted region while keeping the suggested distance to ensure optimal light absorption.

4. Following Treatment:

• Hydration: Maintain adequate hydration to aid in muscle growth and recuperation.

• Nutrition: To support muscle growth and repair, eat a well-balanced diet high in protein and vital nutrients.

• Sleep and relax: To help the body heal and regenerate muscle tissue, make sure you get enough sleep and relax.

Result

• Short-Term: Pain relief right away, a decrease in inflammation and discomfort in the muscles, and a quicker recovery from acute injuries.

Long-term benefits include stronger muscles, a lower chance of overtraining injuries, quicker healing from chronic injuries, and an improvement in overall athletic performance.

Clinical Evidence and Case Studies

1.Muscle Recuperation:

•A study that appeared in "The Journal of Athletic Training" discovered that RLT improved athletes' recuperation after rigorous exercise and greatly decreased muscular soreness.

2. Athletic Injuries:

o Research published in "Photomedicine and Laser Surgery" showed that RLT helped injured athletes recuperate from tendon injuries faster and with less pain and inflammation.

Chapter Eleven

Red Light Therapy for Mood Enhancement and Mental Health

Red light therapy (RLT) is becoming more well-known as a safe, all-natural method of treating mental illness and elevating mood. This area is thought to benefit from it because of its impact on hormone balance, cognitive function, and general well-being. RLT can be used to improve mood and mental health in the following ways:

Mechanisms of Action for Improving Mood and Mental Health

1.Control of Circadian Cycles:

- **Melatonin Production:** By encouraging the body to produce melatonin, the hormone that induces sleep, RLT can assist in regulating the circadian cycles of the body. A better night's sleep is directly associated with happier and more positive mental states.

2. Balance of Neurotransmitters:

- Serotonin Levels: Serotonin is a neurotransmitter linked to emotions of happiness and well-being. RLT may raise serotonin levels. Elevated serotonin levels have been shown to mitigate anxiety and depression symptoms.

3. Decreased Inflammation:

• Reduction of Neuro-inflammation: A number of mental health conditions have been related to chronic inflammation, including neuro-inflammation. The anti-inflammatory properties of RLT can aid in lowering brain inflammation and enhancing mental wellness.

4. Increased Blood Flow:

• Cerebral Circulation: RLT enhances blood flow to the brain, resulting in more effective nutrition and oxygen delivery. Improved cerebral circulation promotes general brain health and cognitive performance.

5. Reducing Stress:

• Cortisol Regulation: The body's main stress hormone, cortisol, may be regulated in part by RLT. A calmer mental state can be encouraged by balanced cortisol levels, which can lower stress and anxiety.

Applications for Improving Mood and Mental Health

1. SAD, or seasonal affective disorder:

• Symptom Alleviation: By mimicking natural sunshine exposure, which is frequently restricted throughout the winter, RLT can help reduce the symptoms of seasonal affective disorder (SAD). Both energy and mood are enhanced by this.

2. Depression

• Mood Improvement: RLT can help reduce inflammation and raise serotonin levels to assist treat depressive symptoms, which in turn improves mood and emotional health.

• Energy Levels: Improved ATP synthesis and mitochondrial activity can raise energy levels, fending off the exhaustion that is frequently linked to depression.

3. Fear:

• Calming Effects: RLT can lessen anxiety and encourage tranquility because of its capacity to control cortisol and increase serotonin synthesis.

• Stress Resilience: Regular RLT

use may increase the body's ability to withstand stress, which will lessen the frequency and severity of anxiety attacks.

4. Disorders of Sleep:

• Better Sleep Quality: RLT can contribute to better sleep quality and length, which is crucial for mental health, by controlling circadian rhythms and encouraging melatonin production.

5. Mental Process:

• Enhanced Brain Function: Memory, attention, and mental clarity can all be supported by improved cerebral circulation and decreased neuro-inflammation.

Use of Red Light Therapy in

Practice for Improving Mood and Mental Health

1.Treatment Duration and Frequency:

• Initial Phase: During the first two to four weeks, RLT can be used everyday to achieve notable improvements in mental health.

• Maintenance Phase: To sustain the positive effects on mental health, treatments can be cut back to three to four times per week after the initial phase.

2. Selection of Device:

• Light therapy lamps: Perfect for full body and facial exposure, these lamps mimic the effects of natural sunlight.

• Handheld devices: Good for

stimulating brain activity in particular locations, such the forehead.

• Wearable Devices: Headbands or spectacles with light therapy are convenient for ongoing treatment.

3. Getting Ready and Using It:

• Timing: To prevent interfering with sleep patterns at night, use RLT in the morning or early afternoon.

• Setting: To maximize the therapeutic benefits, create a cozy and tranquil setting.

4. Following Treatment:

• Hydration: To promote general health and wellbeing, sip lots of water.

• Relaxation: To enhance the relaxing benefits of RLT, use relaxation techniques like deep breathing or meditation.

Result

• **Short-Term:** Higher energy levels, better sleep, less tension and anxiety, and an improved mood.

• **Long-term:** Notable reduction in anxiety and depressive symptoms, improved stress management, increased cognitive function, and general improvement in mental health and wellbeing.

Chapter Twelve

Red light treatment's effects on seasonal affective disorder (SAD)

Depression known as seasonal affective disorder (SAD) usually manifests itself throughout certain seasons of the year, mainly during the winter when there is less exposure to sunlight. Red light treatment (RLT), which mimics the effects of natural sunlight and affects various physiological systems related to mood and energy levels, has demonstrated promise in reducing the symptoms of seasonal affective disorder (SAD).

Mechanisms of Action

1.Control of Circadian Cycles:

• **Production of Melatonin:** RLT aids in the regulation of melatonin synthesis, a hormone that governs sleep-wake cycles. A healthy circadian rhythm can enhance happiness and the quality of sleep.

• **Light Exposure:** Red light exposure, particularly in the morning, can assist in resetting the body's internal clock and lessen the negative effects of winter's decreased natural light.

2. Serotonin Concentrations:

• **Neurotransmitter Balance:** RLT may boost serotonin synthesis, a neurotransmitter linked to emotions of happiness and well-being. Elevated serotonin levels can aid in reducing SAD's depressive symptoms.

3. Improved Circulation of Blood:

• **Cerebral Circulation:** Better oxygen and nutrition delivery to the brain results from increased blood flow, which promotes mood regulation and cognitive function.

4. Decrease in Inflammation:

• **Anti-Inflammatory Effects:** Mental health may be impacted by persistent inflammation. The anti-inflammatory qualities of RLT aid in lowering general inflammation, which may enhance mood and lessen depressive symptoms.

Use of Red Light Therapy in Practice for SAD

1.Treatment Duration and Frequency:

• Daily Sessions: It is advised to utilize RLT every day for 20 to 30 minutes each session, preferably in the morning, in order to effectively control SAD.

• Consistency: To sustain the benefits and avoid symptom recurrence, daily use must be consistent throughout the winter.

2. Selection of Device:

• Light Therapy Lamps: Treatment for SAD is frequently achieved with full-spectrum light therapy lamps. These gadgets are perfect for full-face and body exposure since they can mimic exposure to natural sunshine.

- **Portable Devices**: Full-face lights are generally more successful for treating SAD, although handheld or smaller portable devices can be utilized for targeted exposure.

3. Getting Ready and Using It:

- Timing: The best time of day to reset the circadian cycle and elevate mood is in the morning.
- Setting: To maximize the therapeutic effects, use the therapy in a cozy, well-lit setting.

4. Following Treatment:

- Hydration: Maintain adequate hydration to promote general

health and optimize the therapeutic effect.

• Healthy Habits: Combine RLT with other health-promoting practices, like consistent exercise, a well-balanced diet, and enough sleep.

expected Result

• **Short-Term:** Better mood, more vitality, and higher-quality sleep. After using the product consistently for a few days to a few weeks, users may experience a decrease in depression symptoms.

• **Long-term:** Better mood and energy levels that last throughout the winter, fewer and milder SAD episodes, and an overall increase in wellbeing.

Clinical Evidence and Case Studies

1.Effectiveness of Phototherapy:

• A study that was published in "The American Journal of Psychiatry" discovered that participants' SAD symptoms were greatly improved by light treatment, which included the use of red light. The results of the study demonstrated how crucial morning light exposure is for restoring circadian rhythms and elevating mood.

2.Comparative Research:

• A study that was published in "Psychiatry Research" evaluated light therapy and antidepressants for the treatment of SAD and discovered that light therapy had less negative effects while still being equally effective. Better sleep patterns, more vitality, and an enhanced mood were all mentioned by the participants.

3.Long-Term Advantages:

• A long-term study published in the "Journal of Affective Disorders" showed that consistent use of light therapy during the winter months enhanced quality of life overall and offered long-lasting relief from symptoms of seasonal affective disorder.

Chapter Fourteen

Red Light Therapy for Medical Conditions and Clinical Environments

Owing to its many therapeutic advantages, red light therapy (RLT) is being included into clinical settings and medical treatments more and more. RLT is a tool used by medical experts to treat a variety of illnesses because of its capacity to boost general wellbeing, decrease inflammation, accelerate healing, and relieve pain. RLT is used in clinical settings and medicinal therapies in the following ways:

Mechanisms of Action

1. Improved Cellular Performance:

• **ATP Production:** RLT causes cells to produce more ATP (adenosine triphosphate), which gives cells more energy for internal operations and speeds up healing and regeneration.

2. Anti-Inflammatory Effects:

• Cytokine Modulation: RLT causes an increase in anti-inflammatory cytokines and a decrease in pro-inflammatory cytokines, which contributes to a reduction in inflammation in general.

3. Better Blood Flow: •

Vasodilation: RLT encourages vasodilation, which enhances oxygen supply to tissues and blood flow, promoting healing and lowering pain.

4. Collagen Production: •

Tissue Repair: RLT promotes the synthesis of collagen, which is necessary for the regeneration and repair of tissues, such as tendons, muscles, and skin.

5. Pain Relief: RLT has the ability to alter nerve activity, which lessens the transmission of pain signals and relieves both acute and chronic pain.

Utilizations in Medical Environments

1. Dermatology:

• Wound Healing: By encouraging tissue repair and lowering inflammation, RLT hastens the healing of burns, wounds, and ulcers.

• Skin disorders: By lowering inflammation and encouraging skin regeneration, RLT is used to treat a variety of skin disorders, including as rosacea, eczema, and psoriasis.

• Anti-Aging therapies: By promoting collagen formation, RLT is used to anti-aging therapies to minimize wrinkles and fine lines and enhance skin texture.

2. Orthopedics and Sports Medicine:

• Injury Recovery: By lowering inflammation and encouraging tissue regeneration, RLT is used to treat sports injuries such as tendinitis, ligament sprains, and muscular strains.

• Management of Arthritis: RLT improves joint function and mobility by relieving pain and reducing inflammation in individuals with rheumatoid arthritis and osteoarthritis.

3. Physical Therapy:

• Pain Management: RLT reduces inflammation and modifies nerve activity to relieve pain in disorders such neuropathy, persistent back pain, and neck discomfort.

• Rehabilitation: By promoting cellular repair processes and boosting blood flow, RLT aids in the recovery from musculoskeletal injuries.

4. Dental Care:

• Oral Inflammation: RLT facilitates healing and lessens inflammation in gingivitis, periodontitis, and following oral procedures.

• Pain Relief: RLT relieves pain in the mouth, such as headaches and temporomandibular joint (TMJ) issues.

5. Mental Health:

• Mood Enhancement: By boosting serotonin production and controlling circadian rhythms, RLT is used to improve mood and lessen the symptoms of anxiety and despair.

• Sleep Disorders: RLT is helpful for people with insomnia or other sleep disorders since it helps control sleep-wake cycles and enhances the quality of sleep.

Usefulness in Medical Procedures

1. Device Selection:

• Professional equipment: To provide accurate and efficient treatments, clinical settings employ powerful RLT equipment, such as tailored light arrays and full-body panels.

• Portable Devices: Handheld, smaller devices are utilized for focused treatments, giving clinicians more freedom to target particular problem areas.

2. Protocols for Treatment:

• Frequency and Duration:
Depending on the ailment being
treated, different treatment
methods apply. Sessions typically
last for 10 to 30 minutes and
occur two to five times a week on
average.

• Customization: Treatment plans
are tailored to each patient's
needs, the severity of their
ailment, and how well they
respond to treatment.

3. Setting Up the Patient:

• Clean Treatment Area: To
optimize light penetration, make
sure the treatment area is clear
of lotions and other obstructions.

• Precautionary Steps: When administering facial treatments, both patients and professionals should wear the proper eye protection.

4. After-Treatment Care:

• Nutrition and Hydration: To aid the body's healing processes, patients should be encouraged to consume a balanced diet and stay hydrated.

• Follow-Up: Scheduling routine follow-up visits to assess progress and modify treatment plans as necessary.

Chapter Fifteen

Red Light Therapy: Consumer Applications and At-Home Devices

Red light therapy, or RLT, is becoming more and more well-liked among people who want to enhance their fitness and health without leaving their homes. Technological developments have increased the affordability, accessibility, and usability of RLT devices. An overview of at-home technology and its uses in daily living is provided below:

Types of Red Light Therapy Devices for Home Use

1. Handheld Devices:

• Described as small, lightweight gadgets that are intended to target particular body parts.

• Uses: Perfect for addressing small skin regions, focused muscle rehabilitation, and localized discomfort.

2. LED Panels:

• Characteristics: Bigger panels that can encompass a greater portion of the face or torso.

• Uses: Excellent for full-body treatments, skin renewal, and general well-being.

3. Wearable Devices:

• Definition: Applies to items like belts, wraps, and masks that are intended to be worn on the body.

• Applications: Ideal for continual massage of the face, knees, or back.

4. Light Therapy lights:

• Characteristics: Fixed lights that offer a wide range of light.

• Applications: Frequently used to treat seasonal affective disorder (SAD) and improve mood.

Red light therapy applications for consumers

1. Anti-Aging and Skin Care:

• Wrinkle Reduction: RLT promotes the formation of collagen, which lessens the visibility of wrinkles and fine lines.

• Acne Treatment: Promotes cleaner skin by assisting in the reduction of inflammation and bacteria linked to acne.

• Scar Reduction: By improving cellular repair, this technique speeds up healing and lessens the visibility of scars.

2. Handling Pain:

• Joint Pain: Treats ailments including arthritis by reducing inflammation and relieving pain.

• Muscle Soreness: Reduces
soreness during physical activity
or exercise and speeds up
recovery.

• Chronic Pain: Offers relief from
long-term ailments like
fibromyalgia and lower back pain.

3. Mood Improvement and Mental Well-Being:

• Seasonal Affective Disorder
Treatment: Reduces symptoms of
the disorder by simulating
sunlight.

• Anxiety and Depression:
Regulates circadian rhythms and
increases serotonin synthesis,

which elevates mood and lowers stress.

• Sleep Improvement: Melatonin synthesis and circadian rhythms are regulated to promote better quality sleep.

4. Recuperation and Fitness:

• Muscle Recovery: Boosts ATP synthesis in cells, hastening the healing of muscles after exercise.

• Sports Injuries: Promotes healing of sprains and strains by reducing inflammation.

• Enhancement of Performance: Consistent use can promote muscular growth and enhance sports performance.

Chapter Sixteen

Useful Advice about Red Light Therapy Equipment at Home

1. Device Choice:

• Goal: Select a gadget according to its intended usage (e.g., handheld for focused therapy, panels for full-body use).

• Quality: Seek out FDA-approved products with favorable feedback and demonstrated effectiveness.

2. Usage Instructions:

• Frequency: For best effects, adhere to the manufacturer's instructions, which call for doing this three to five times a week.

- Duration: Depending on the treatment region and equipment, sessions typically last 10 to 20 minutes.

3. Safety Measures:

- Eye Protection: To avoid possible eye damage during face treatments, wear goggles or make sure your eyes are closed.

- Skin Sensitivity: To test skin sensitivity, begin with shorter sessions and progressively increase exposure.

4. Upkeep and Handling:

- Cleaning: To maintain longevity and hygiene, clean the equipment on a regular basis in accordance with the manufacturer's recommendations.

• Storage: To avoid damage, keep the gadget in a dry, cold place.

Anticipated outcomes and advantages

• **Short-Term:** Feel better right away, less pain and inflammation, and higher-quality sleep.

• **Long-Term:** Better mental health, quicker muscular recovery, enhanced skin appearance, and long-lasting pain relief.

User Stories and Testimonials

1. Skin Care: After a few weeks of regular use, users report measurable improvements in skin texture and less acne.

2. Pain Management:

• Significant relief from chronic pain conditions and increased joint mobility are reported by many users.

3. Mood and Sleep:

• Following consistent RLT sessions, individuals with SAD and insomnia report feeling happier and having better sleep habits.

Chapter Seventeen

Including Red Light Therapy in Everyday Activities

Red light therapy (RLT) can be easily incorporated into everyday routines to improve general health and wellbeing. Here's how you may easily incorporate RLT into several facets of your life:

Creating a Schedule

1. Always Be Consistent:

• Regular Schedule: Whether it's in the morning, afternoon, or evening, decide on a regular time each day for your RLT sessions. Maintaining consistency improves the therapy's overall effects.

• Daily or Weekly Use: For best effects, use RLT daily or many times per week, depending on your objectives and the manufacturer's recommendations.

2. Length of Session:

• Short Sessions: As your body adjusts, start with shorter sessions, about 10-15 minutes, and progressively extend to 20-30 minutes.

• Timing: While evening sessions might promote rest and recuperation, morning sessions can assist balance circadian cycles and increase vitality.

Morning Schedule

1. Increasing Mood and Energy:

• Wake-Up Ritual: Include a little RLT session in your morning regimen to aid in mental and physical awakening. When having breakfast or reading, use a light treatment lamp or panel.

• Morning Exercise: To improve muscular function and recuperation, use RLT either before or after your morning workout.

2. Skin Care Schedule:

• Preparing the Skin: To improve skin texture and lessen indications of aging, incorporate a

10-minute RLT session into your morning skincare routine.

• Complementary Products: To improve absorption and effectiveness, apply your skincare products following the RLT session.

Midday Schedule

1. Rest Periods:

• Reducing Stress: To improve attention and lower stress, use a light therapy lamp or a portable RLT gadget during work breaks.

• Desk Setup: Throughout the workday, use a small RLT device that you place on your desk for brief sessions.

2. Pain Relief:

• Targeted Treatment: Apply RLT in the middle of the day to relieve any arising pain or discomfort, such as stiff joints from extended sitting or back pain.

Evening Schedule

1. Relaxation and Recovery:

• Post-Exercise Recovery: Use RLT to aid in muscle recovery and lessen discomfort following nighttime workouts.

• Wind-Down Routine: As part of your evening relaxation routine, use RLT to help you wind down and get ready for a restful night's sleep.

2. Enhancing Sleep:

• Use RLT Before Bedtime: A quick RLT session one to two hours before to bedtime will assist control the synthesis of melatonin and enhance the quality of your sleep.

• Sleep Environment: To create a relaxing, healing atmosphere that promotes sleep, keep an RLT device in your bedroom.

Combining This Wellness Practice with Others

1. Mindfulness and Meditation:

• Enhanced Meditation: To improve mental clarity and

relaxation during mindfulness or meditation sessions, apply RLT.

• Calming properties: RLT's calming properties can enhance your meditation practice and foster a calmer atmosphere.

2. Yoga and Stretching:

• Pre- or Post-Yoga: Use RLT before to or following yoga sessions to increase overall benefits, decrease muscle tension, and improve flexibility.

3. Complementary Therapies:

• Massage Therapy: To promote relaxation, lessen tense muscles, and increase circulation, combine RLT with massage therapy.

• Aromatherapy: Combine RLT with aromatherapy to create a multisensory relaxing experience that enhances both physical and mental health.

Advice for a Successful Integration

1. Convenient Placement & Ease of Access: To promote frequent use, keep your RLT devices in easily accessible places like your living room, workstation, or by your bed.

• Portability: For ease and adaptability in various environments, use lightweight, portable equipment.

2. Personalization

• Customized Sessions: You can design your RLT sessions to address particular issues, like improving your mood, relieving pain, or taking care of your skin.

• Modifiable Settings: To personalize your treatments, use gadgets with modifiable timer and intensity settings.

3. Knowledge and Sensitization:

• Stay Informed: To optimize the advantages of RLT, stay current on the most recent findings and suggestions.

• Monitor Progress: Keep tabs on your development and modify your regimen as necessary in response to your body's reaction to the therapy.